'Shit Yours

#syst

By

Joseph McNally

<u>Disclaimer</u>

While all the events in this book are true, I do not accept any personal responsibility for the consequences of any individual's actions after reading this.

Basically, please don't shit yourself to death. We have only just got over the last three court cases.

The purpose of this document is to share my experiences while poking a little bit of fun at myself.

I am glad if you find the information contained useful but that was not my intention.

Finally, thank you for purchasing this book!

Introduction

I have always eaten well ("well" meaning I am a human dustbin, it just sounds nicer) which has caused my weight to fluctuate up and down over the years and I kind of blame my Nan for that.

When my Mum was at university and Dad was working away we would always go to my Nan's house for dinner after school. You would walk in her front door at 16:01, be screamed at because you were one minute late, dinner was on the table and as a result ruined. Even though it was the buses fault and not yours, you were late! You even said you wouldn't get to hers until after 4pm anyway.

She would then put enough food for five people on a plate in front of you and you had no choice but to eat this food or forever be trapped at the dinner table. This is all while Nan ate only one potato and a slice of meat because she wasn't a big eater.

Whatever she gave us, we ate it! We never took prisoners. We never gave in. We even tried to become vegetarians when Mum did it for a bet with her friend.

"Nan, I'm a vegetarian!"

"No, you're not!"

slams potato cooked three ways on a plate in front you

We completely lost any comprehension as to what portion control was. "You must eat everything on your plate!" was her mantra and it is something I have taken with me all my life.

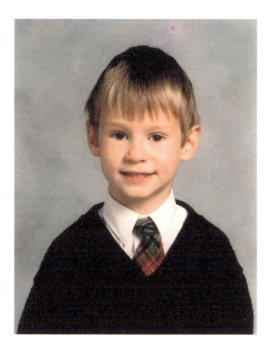

This was me before I got fat. Please forgive the haircut, we were poor.

Now my weight had never really bothered me to be totally honest in the past, but it was only after talking to my friend about dressing up for the next time we went to the Rocky Horror Picture Show at the theatre I thought I am never going to fit into my H&M corset as it currently stands. What was I going to do about it?

I contemplated sewing two H&M corsets together but that would mean 1) going back to the shop and being stared at by the shop assistant like I was a weirdo…again and 2) effort. I am a lazy person so that was a no go. I could have paid Nan to have made it in hindsight, but I'll do that next time.

Anyway, back to my original point. Lose weight of course and make it fit, but how?!

This was a photo of me back in 2012 when I hit 17 stone! Just before I tried 'Weight Watchers'.

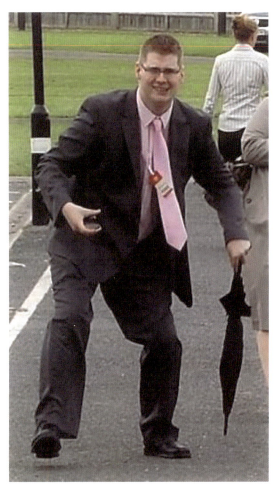

Quite a revolting photo really. My weight has greatly fluctuated over the last ten years.

Below is a picture of me in Mexico back in November 2015, before I started this journey. Now I cannot remember if this is at the start of the holiday or after I had eaten the equivalent of a small herd of cattle and got seriously sunburnt, but you get the idea. I had a cute and chubby face don't you think?

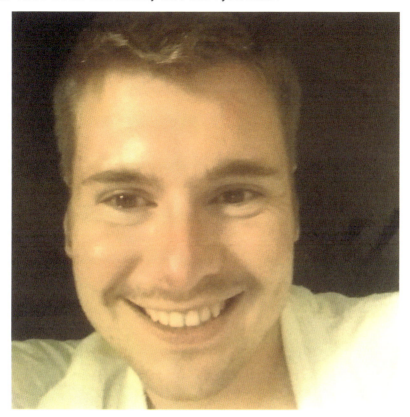

This was my weight and BMI at the same time. I needed to decide how to lose the weight.

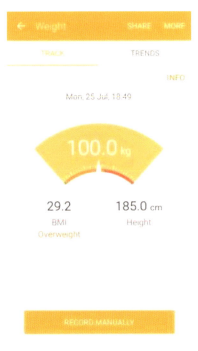

Now, I am seriously a very lazy person when it comes to any form of physical activity. All my hobbies can in fact be done lying down or via the internet, preferably both.

I am not a gym bunny and I am not willing to make ANY time to go to the gym so this scuppered the idea of going to the gym to lose weight. I had tried 'Weight Watchers' to some success losing one and half stone back in 2012 however I did not feel this was right approach for me this time around. I never stayed for the meetings in fact and basically paid five pounds per week for someone else to weigh me and judge me. This was something I could have done at home in mirror.

I needed something new, something different, something that screamed Joseph. When it hit me. What were the two things I am good at, talking and making shit.

So, I started looking at diet and exercise plans on the internet to get a feel for what was out there. Obviously while eating some chocolate for brain food. I was rocking my new hairdo at the time.

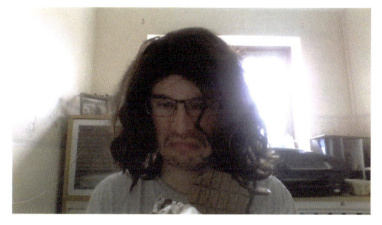

You can tell by my facial expressions I was not impressed by what I found. Nothing tailored to people like me.

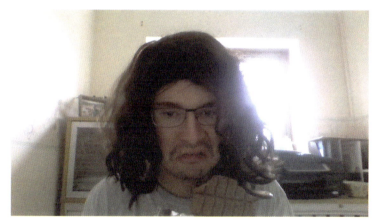

But there was something I did find which was very interesting, which was chilli peppers can help you lose weight.

Now this was exciting. I love chilli peppers. I love hot food. In fact, I tried the world's hottest chilli pepper while writing this book which at the time was the 'Carolina Reaper' because I love the heat so much. It does always amaze me how I can sweat so much out of the sides of my head when I have hot food.

I started thinking, could I lose weight eating lots of chilli as part of a normal routine? What would the side effects be?

I remember as a kid going to the cinema with my friends, deciding on what film to watch and before going in buying lots of overpriced snacks which at the time required your parents to re-mortgage their home to raise the funds. Which ironically hasn't changed. As I was thinking I was the dog's bollocks I would always get the nachos, with hot cheese sauce and have it covered, I mean COVERED in green jalapenos.

However, because I was unseasoned I wouldn't even chew the jalapenos, I would just swallow them sandwiched between two nachos to try and avoid the searing pain in my mouth and work towards that satisfaction of knowing I had beaten the tray.

The next morning, as you can imagine that sweet satisfaction turned to seer regret as the 'Poor Man's Colon Clean' (trademark the Justin Household, 2004) took hold and my bowels attempted to emigrate from my body. No amount of wet toilet paper could alleviate the pain in which I was enduring at the time.

The Justin household has since bought me these soothing and moisturising toilet wipes to ease any future regrets.

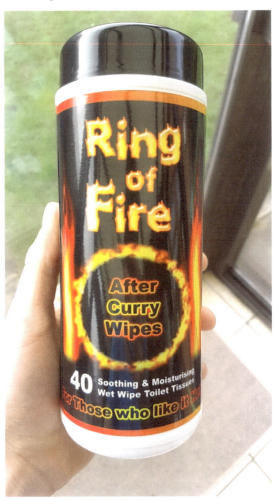

These memories ensured I was truly aware of what would happen if I started a diet very heavily incorporating hot chilli peppers. However, to lose the weight I was ready to make that sacrifice.

The "Science"

There is some loose "science" that this concept/diet call it what you will is based on.

Chillies are high in vitamin C and contain more vitamin C than oranges! Vitamin C is needed by the body to produce white blood cells which fight unwelcome visitors in the body helping to keep you well.

Chillies contain beta-carotene which the body converts to vitamin A. Vitamin A is essential for ensuring that your immune system works efficiently and protects you from illness and infection.

Most importantly they include capsaicin. This is the chemical which reacts with the nerve endings in your mouth and producing the famous fiery burn. Capsaicin can help to reduce inflammation in the body and increase the number of antibodies in your body meaning fewer infections.

It is believed that chillies can temporarily increase your body's metabolism by between 5% to 15% (dependent on who you speak to) after eating. Which when coupled with exercise can lead to greater weight loss results. It takes about 30 mins for the metabolism to be impacted so exercise should be done 30 mins after consuming the chillies.

While this plan does not include exercise, this is a useful fact to know.

Spicy food can also increase the feeling of being full after a meal which can help people to control their food intake better which is a key to weight loss.

Spicy food can also cause you to heavily sweat and moan really loud while eating, bit like…..

Feels like a super food to me!

Going Balls Deep

So, with the commitment made to lose weight and the "science" behind me it was time to undertake the journey.

Now I decided that Monday evenings were going to be my weigh in day. I have no logic behind why. I think it was just this was the first day after I started my diet. However, it is essential for consistency that you only weigh yourself once a week at the same time. I know people who (and have done it myself) weigh themselves daily and just depress the hell out of themselves. 3lb up, then 4lb down, then 5lb up, you get the idea, but my hot tip has to be "I never weigh myself unless I've done a poo!" It could be the difference between losing weight for that week and putting on weight.

My next step was what hot sauce do I want to use? Now when I'm talking hot sauce I am not talking lemon and herb from your favourite fried chicken shop or sweet chilli sauce. I am talking habanero, ghost chilli, scotch bonnet, extra hot, tear inducing pain sauces. This plan has no exercise so there must be some kind of pain!

The hot sauce is the first part to the success of this plan.

These sauces come in all shapes and sizes with a variety of different, fear inducing names but the key is you must choose a hot sauce which is going to push you, but not starting so hot you effectively ruin every meal as well as your insides and taste buds.

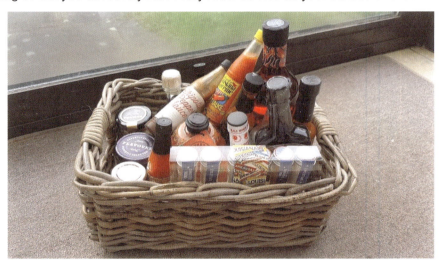

As I regularly eat chillies and hot sauce my starting point was relatively high hence I could dive straight into the above. A good starting point for you might be jalapeno, which for someone who does not eat hot food on a regular basis packs a punch.

Your body adapts to the fiery heat of the chilli and over time you will build up a tolerance which means you can and need to go to the next level and the good news there is ALWAYS another level. Chilli growers around the world are always trying to cross breed and invent new hot chilli, and this is part of the reason why the world's hottest chilli is always changing as times passes by.

What is good about your body building a tolerance to the heat of the chilli is you can start to really savour the flavour of the sauce and chilli you are eating. People do not realise that chillies all have their own distinct, unique flavours ranging from bitter through to sweet and fruity.

I started with some ghost chilli sauces and this was because I started this diet in January 2016 I was using all the hot sauces my family and friends had bought me for Christmas due to me already having a reputation for hot food. You can always tell it is January as all the Weight Watchers yoghurts are sold out in ASDA.

The second part to the success of this plan is that this plan is a low carbohydrate diet.

Hot Sauce + Low Carbohydrate Diet = Sexy New You

I really scaled back on carbohydrate effectively eliminating it from my diet. It became more a treat than a staple in my diet especially for the first three to six months when I lost most of my weight. Any carbohydrate was limited to white rice or sweet potatoes and mostly consumed if I was intending on drinking alcohol that day. I did not eat bread or potatoes if it could be avoided. The basis of all my meals consisted of protein like meat and egg accompanied with if possible lots of fresh vegetables and salad.

Chicken + Egg + Hot sauce = Heaven

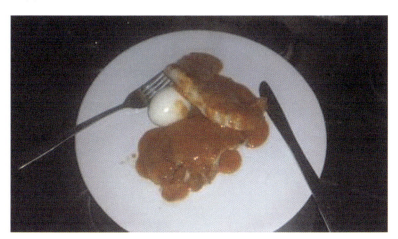

This shift to a high protein based diet has resulted in me developing an obsession for eggs. I love eggs! I will now have at least two eggs per day, every day (with hot sauce of course).

Eggs are a little bit of a super hero. They are cheap, packed full of protein and vitamins including D, B6, B12, zinc, iron and copper. They are like little complete meals all wrapped in their own shell. Just don't eat the shell. Eggs are also good at keeping you feeling full which is what protein does so they can help to stop you snacking during the day and maximise your weight loss plan saving potentially up to 400 calories per day based on some studies.

My favourite breakfast nicknamed the 'Mexican breakfast' – eggs, toast, fresh chilli and hot sauce!

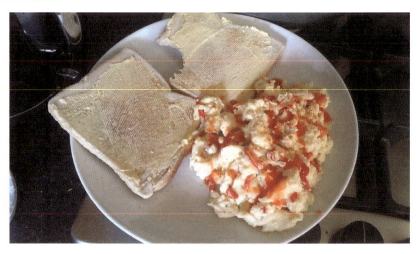

I have shared later a basic guide for your daily diet plan which can be amended to suit your needs and requirements. It gives you a limit on how many calories per day you want to consume and it is because of this limit it started making me think about what I was eating and the nutritional content in that food.

I wanted to get the biggest bang for my buck and maximise my daily limit, so I would swap food items for lower calories alternatives or completely avoid high calorie, fatty foods reserving them as a special treat. What helped to make this plan easy for me was this food swapping and resistance to high calorie, fatty foods became a habit and part of my routine making it easier to lose the weight.

'Shit Yourself Thin' TM Starter Pack

12 x Toilet Rolls

1 x Nappy Rash Cream

3 x Packs of Wet Wipes

2 x Scotch Bonnet Sauce

1 x Pack Fresh Birds Eye Chillies

Quote CANTSITDOWN29

Get yours now at your nearest supermarket

One of the unexpected advantages to the #syst plan was that the dog no longer begs me for food, since she has learnt that hot sauce and dogs do not mix! Bless her.

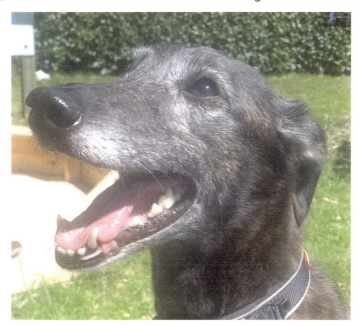

What I did really enjoy about this plan, was due to the calorie savings that you were making during the week you could have heavy weekends every now and then and still enjoy yourself. However, portion size is SO important during the whole week and weekend like eating seven jacket potatoes is not needed, seriously.

While I was doing the #syst plan I did get to finally try the 'Deep Fried Mars Bar' and it was amazing! Even if it did look like a deep-fried turd. Which shows you can still really treat yourself if you want too. I did kind of feel a weeks' worth of hard work was being un-done but you really must try it. So, warm and sticky. A well-deserved treat.

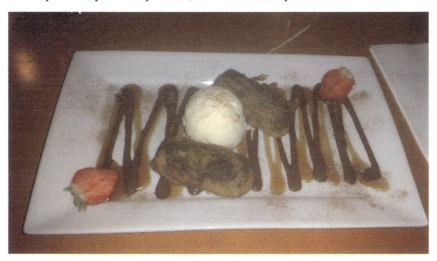

Alcohol

Drinking alcohol can be a nightmare for people trying to slim down due to alcohol being full of sugar and sugar meaning lots of extra, empty calories. People usually get caught out and do not count the calories they are drinking. Most diet plans encourage you to reduce or stop drinking alcohol.

The 'Shit Yourself Thin' plan makes an exception to this and encourages you to have a good time as long as you choose the right alcohol.

The trick is to stick to spirits like rum and gin with diet mixers or light sparkling wines like Prosecco to really limit the calorie intake when you're drinking. Avoid beer and cider which are both carbohydrate heavy drinks and fruit juices. Cocktails can be bad for calories due to the amount of sugary fruit juices that are in them.

Another way to reduce the number of calories you are consuming is to use smaller drinking vessels. These mini copper mugs are great!

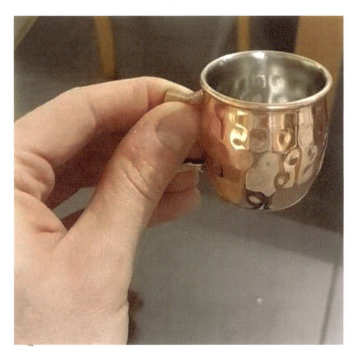

Everyone knows the best cocktails have the least amount of ingredients, ideally with all those ingredients being alcohol. The favourite one being the Margarita!

As one of my favourite past times and hobbies is making and drinking cocktails when I landed in Seattle–Tacoma International Airport back in September 2016 and saw this sign I knew I had come to a place where they had got their priorities right. Always booze then food.

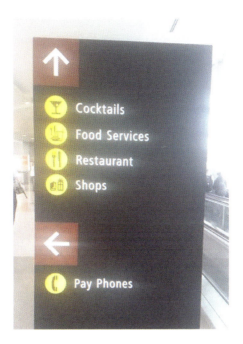

But it was during a visit to New York, the week earlier that I discovered an amazing jalapeno margarita. The bar had soaked loads of green jalapenos in a huge vat of silver tequila which gave the cocktail a warm kick with every sip and this gave me an idea for when I got home!

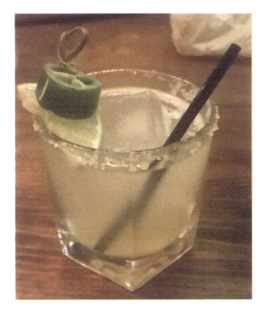

Now not to be one to be out done AND keeping in the spirit of 'Shit Yourself Thin' I decided to have a go at making my own chilli tequila. The logic being I could enjoy my favourite cocktail in the world mixed with fierce heat, vitamins, minerals and metabolism increasing qualities of chilli. It would be like the cocktail version of Slim Fast. Nothing could be better or go wrong.

So, I made two batches.

Batch 1 – Silver tequila mixed with the standard red chillies you get in the supermarket. Usually in packs of three and medium heat (below)

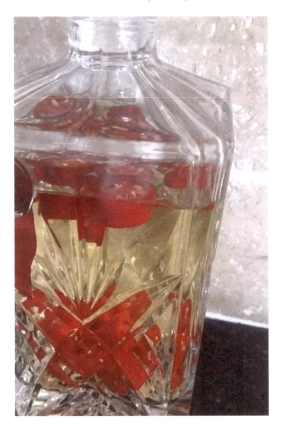

This was nice, the chilli added a bit of warmth to the drink and gave it a bit of colour. However, it was nothing mind blowing and I had to add a lot of red chilli to really get some heat from the drink. Not ideal for my perfect cocktail.

Batch 2 – Silver tequila mixed with Scotch Bonnet chilli

This was something else! 'Fire Water' is the only term I can use to describe what it felt like to drink it, I basically shit myself instantaneously on the first sip since it was so hot and I had to run to the loo.

But this was exactly what I wanted, fierceness in a glass. I made several batches of it and reserved them for special friends or enemies.

Now because this was too hot to drink in its pure liquid form I had to dilute it and I wanted to make a drink that was cold to drink but had a hot feeling in the mouth.

I started by making a normal margarita with my standard recipe:

50ml Tequila

25ml Cointreau

Half a Fresh Lime

25ml Sugar Syrup

Mixed and shaken over ice

Served in a salt rimmed glass

Scale up as required for bigger cocktails

For the Tequila I used 50ml of the 'Fire Water' I had created.

It just didn't work. It was way too hot! Your lips were burning with every sip. It made your eyes sting as you lifted it to your face. It made your stomach cramp, hurt and ache. It would had been great if you needed to relieve constipation or a cold instantaneously.

My next brain wave was to mix 25ml 'Fire Water' and 25ml standard Tequila and this time it worked perfectly. An ice-cold drink, with a fiery and citrus kick the 'Of Fire and Ice' was born!

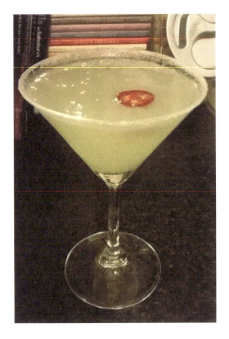

Of Fire and Ice - The Slimmer's Dream

Eat, shit, wipe, repeat!

I have pulled together an example day of what the 'Shit Yourself Thin' diet looks like.

This is what I would base my day's food and calorie intake on.

There is SO much variety you can add into this so please only use this as a guide but do remember this is a LOW carbohydrate diet.

You need to aim for around 1,500 calories per day. I know this is low for both men (RDA 2,500) and women (RDA 2,000) but I never said this would be easy.

Your calorie intake may vary based on alcohol consumption, finger buffets (my one Achilles heel), your commitment and sheer stubbornness.

Typical day:

BREAKFAST:

Choose from:

1 slice of toasted bread, knob of low fat margarine, one large egg, cooked tomatoes

Or

Two large eggs, two rashers of turkey bacon, mushrooms, cooked tomatoes

LUNCH:

Choose from:

Nothing (your trying to lose weight!)

Or

Go Ahead Biscuits (x 3)

Or

1 bag of crisps (150 calories or less)

Plus

Any Fruit (up to 2 pieces) – I like apples and pears!

DINNER:

Grilled meat - choice from chicken/turkey breasts (x2), turkey/low fat pork sausages (x4), rump steak (8oz), white fish (x2 fillets)

Serve with a large mixed salad and low fat dressing and roasted sweet potato and/or other vegetables

Weight Watchers Fat Free Yoghurt and/or Ice Lolly (100 calories or lower)

SNACK:

Are you really going to ask?!

I would expect during this plan basing it on the above skeleton for you to lose between 2 to 3lb per week.

Mishaps

'Shit Yourself Thin' isn't all plain sailing boys and girls. I have had my share of touches of cloth.

Italic text represents a social media update.

"Is it wrong I am smearing yoghurt on my face to stop the burning?!"

I have now learnt the answer is <u>no</u> it is not wrong. Dairy products are great for reducing the burn of any hot sauce or chilli as milk contains casein which effectively binds with the capsaicin in the chilli's and takes it away. It must be mammal milk though so my sister's breast milk could have been an option if I was desperate. I am glad to say I was not. I recommend beef milk but readers' choice. The only down side with dairy products and smearing them all over the affected area is it is not pretty when it starts to warm up and run everywhere. It can make for embarrassing social situations, especially in public forums.

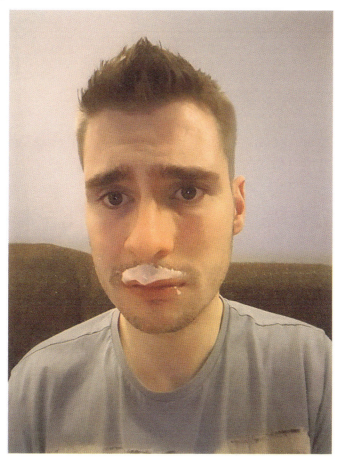

"Scrambled egg gone wrong. Looks like vomit."

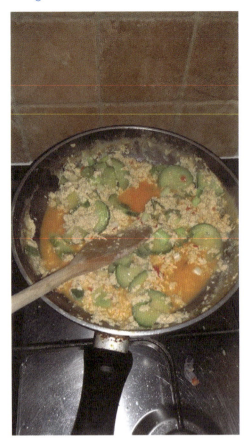

This made me sad. I was hungover and really wanted some eggs (did I say I love eggs?!) and thought it would be a great idea to mix in all the leftovers from the fridge, so cucumber, onion etc. What I ended up was a frying pan of vomit. Amazingly it appears to have carrot in it. I didn't put in any carrot!

I will admit I did eat it. It was that or starving! It was the water in the cucumber that ruined everything. Great for cocktails, bad for eggs!

"I farted in a zipped up long coat. The fart travelled up to my face. I farted in my own face."

I was walking the dog one Sunday morning in the field near my house and the coat I was wearing was too big for me having slimmed down. Too big from a length and width point of view. The coat hung past my pert bottom. I decided to let one go into the wind while we were walking thinking it would be fine. The long coat stopped the gas and smell travelling anywhere but up towards my hooded head and face. It was too late before I realised what was happening.

"My left hand is now too skinny and as a result I have lost one of my rings down the sink!"

"Lost my rings – two, one in a hotel and another hungover on the sofa."

As I lost weight with the #syst plan my fingers unexpectedly got skinner. Which did amaze me to be honest. The three rings I wore started to become loose on my hands as the plan continued. To the point, I could shake my hand and it would ring like a musical instrument as the rings on one hand all hit each other.

I unfortunately managed to lose one ring that my partner bought me in St Maarten down a sink in a hotel just innocently washing my hands with soap. The other fell off when I was sitting on the sofa minding my own business watching a film. I only found it weeks later, after I had to tell him I'd lost another one. I recently lost my engagement ring either at work or walking the dog. So be careful!

Occasionally even now I will be very animatingly talking to someone with my hands and a ring will fly off and hit someone or something.

"You become addicted! Everything tastes bland!"

"Disappointed by the breakfast I made. I knew no hot sauce would be a mistake."

Chillies contain endorphins which can cause your central nervous system to give you a bit of a 'high'. People become addicted or hooked on hot food and chilli's and as you build up your tolerance you end up in this vicious circle where food without it tastes bland and boring so you up the ante. My little sister messaged me when I moved out my parents' house years ago saying ever since you left all my food tastes bland. I took all the hot sauces with me.

"My ring is a mess again."

One of the major issues with eating lots of hot sauce on a low carbohydrate diet is you kind of lose the ability to make a solid stool, something I always took for granted before. Therefore, I recommend you carry with you at all times a pack of wet wipes in case they are needed. I was talking to a colleague the other day at work about the hot wings he had made the night before and how he had one messy poo that morning. I said smugly I bet you wish you had a bidet now!

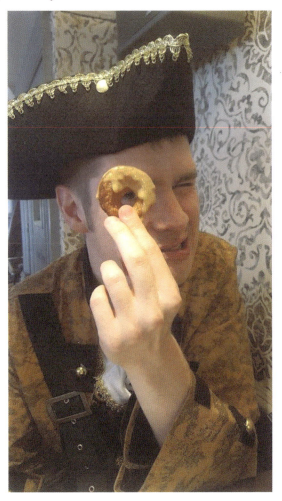

"Still has horrific wind. Going to have to find out what's stuck up there."

I never did find out. To the disappointment of everyone around me and most of St Albans.

"Ok. Ok. Three whole chilli's and hot sauce for dinner is too much. I am full of regret."

It is easy to eat too much chilli for two reasons:

1) you over estimated your tolerance and ability

2) you're showing off (something I have done a few times)

Years ago, Mum and Dad were away and I was staying with my Nan and we went to the pub for some cheeky drinks. I was fifteen/sixteen I think. It was a Saturday night and before the smoking ban so it was busy. One of my Dad's friends was there with a bottle of Tabasco sauce and spurred on with my experiences with the nachos and jalapenos at the cinema (mentioned before) I was emboldened.

"Who wants to try some sauce?!"

"I will." – I screamed.

I grabbed the bottle and begin to pour it down my neck to the horror of those in the pub around me. I stopped and looked at them all after for a brief second before a blood curdling scream radiated out of my mouth and I ran into the toilet with a bright red face.

My Nan didn't realise what had happened except for seeing me run into the toilet with a fire in my mouth. She burst into the men's toilet after me thinking I had done drugs and was dying (always a melodramatic family). She scolded me repeatedly while I was face down in a sink of cold water. Once I was in a better state I had the embarrassment factor of walking back into the pub and sitting down in front of everyone, a broken man.

This was only one time I have embarrassed myself under estimating my tolerance.

It happened again years later. Mum went to Wales to see her friend and bought me back a Chocolate Habanero sauce for me as a gift/punishment (jury is still out). Apparently, it was the hottest one in the shop she smugly told me. It even had a voodoo doll on the label so this should have been a red flag for me, but it wasn't.

"Ah thanks Mum, I'll try it now!" – I chimed.

I walked over the kitchen drawer, grabbed a dessert spoon, filled it up and swallowed the sauce all in one go.

The burn was intense and I felt it burning my mouth and oesophagus as it travelled slowly down however, as I am pro I showed no facial expression or pain (played it cool) and then decided to make my way home with the dog.

I said goodbye to Mum and Dad, got in the car, started driving home. The pain was gradually building in intensity and by now my eyes were streaming and I couldn't concentrate on driving the car. "Can I make it home, can I make it?!" I panickedly thought. Ten minutes till home no problems could I do it?!

The answer was a resounding no! I spun the car around and sped back to my parents. Mounted the kerb while parking. Ran towards the front door leaving the dog in the car wondering what the hell was going on. I bashed on the door as I was in too much pain to try and open it with my own key. As Mum opened the door and I barged past her and ran straight for the fridge. I grabbed several yoghurts and started eating them as fast as possible. Mum was in a panic as she didn't know what was going on.

I was starting to get severe shakes and felt panicked which was alarming and I was concerned about going into a state of shock. I stood there shaking looking pathetic with my Mum glaring back at me judgementally in the dining room when a very calm and intellectual voice popped into my head.

"After everything we have achieved I never thought it would end like this. God, you're stupid." – my brain

Thankfully the yoghurt had started to take effect and the pain and shaking subsided. I just sat quietly in the dining room trying to recover my strength and composure to the chorus of "Stupid boy." I had NO intention of EVER doing that again.

ALWAYS respect the chilli.

"Was coughing so hard in bed last night, I nearly shit myself!"

The one good thing I found with the #syst diet was that my immune system did not seem to get run down due to the vitamins and health benefits associated with the chilli. This is unlike others I know who have tried different diets over the years and found themselves always under the weather or falling ill.

I did have a near miss though when suffering a chronic cough. I coughed and my body mistook the movement. Had to climb out of bed and make it to the loo while fully clenched. Made the Olympics seem a doddle.

Overheard in Spanish, the maintenance man phoning for help, "Some dirty bastard has blocked the toilet and we don't know what to do?!"

Ok, this one is not real, but I was on holiday drinking rum watching two maintenance guys arguing in Spanish over something and it seemed fun to add a voice over.

"Vindaloo poo number 3 #poormanscolonclean #syst"

I had a curry at my parents from the local takeaway. I had it at 6pm and was already on the loo regretting it about 10/11pm. I had not even been to bed which was annoying!

I find vindaloo's and hot curry's a great alarm clock. Have one before bed and I guarantee you'll be up at 4am. Those stomach cramps work like clockwork.

Never miss that important business meeting or presentation again!

"Ghost Chilli Poltergeist have become a regular occurrence. We wouldn't mind, but he has a tendency for latex."

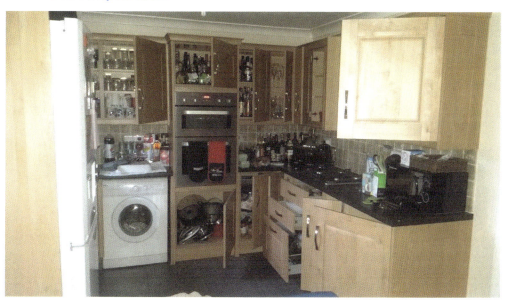

This was a bit tedious. We bought a chilli sauce back from our holiday in Mexico and managed to bring back an Aztec spirit who loved opening every kitchen cupboard and latex gloves. Very odd. We named him Itzcóatl.

"Whenever I come here there is always a dirty bastard ahead of me!"

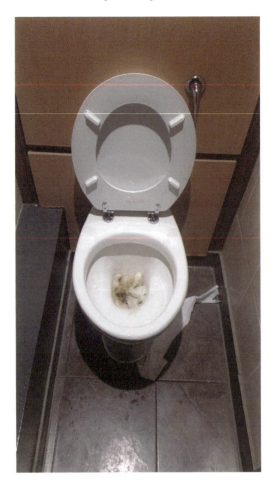

This is like my pet hate! Walking into the loo after someone else and they have not had the decency to clean up properly. I end up getting embarrassed in case others think it's me, cleaning the whole toilet and then make a point of pointing it out to everyone else in the toilet I didn't make the smell.

I once worked in an office in Milton Keynes where someone had done a poo NEXT to the toilet. Why?! Did they fall off?

Really one of life's great mysteries.

"Nearly died but California Reaper Hot Wings done!"

I was in Ireland visiting some family and my cousins wanted to go out to Kilkenny for lunch. They insisted we went to this restaurant who were famous for their chicken wings, which was fine with me because I LOVE chicken wings, especially spicy ones.

So, we went to the restaurant and I was sitting there looking all fabulous flicking through the menu admiring the choice of different types of wings when one caught my eye. 'Loco Caliente' they were called. Having made my choice, I gave my order to the waitress.

"Can I have the Loco Caliente wings please?" I said smiling.

"Are you sure? They are hot." replied the waitress in a fed up, monotone voice.

"Yeah, that's fine!" I said. "I love hot food!"

"But sir. These are REALLY hot, I've never seen anyone finish them."

"It's OK. I'm a professional. Bring them out!"

The waitress did not realise, but she had issued me with a challenge and being the overconfident twat that I am, I insisted that I be filmed eating these wings, so I could demonstrate my abilities to others.

I found out online after my lunch that someone had referred to these wings as "inedible" and I can completely relate to that now however at the time I did not take heed to the waitress' warnings and soon arrived a massive bowl of wings.

Now I'm not sure if I was lucky with the size of the bowl, because you usually only get three or four wings for a starter or if the waitress was trying to teach me a lesson, but there was only one option but to jump in.

I picked up the first wing, taking care to ensure I did not touch any parts of my face and started to the eat the wing. The heat immediately hit me. It was a searing heat. Beads of sweat started to form at the top of my head, but I continued to gobble it down. I proceeded to eat through wings two and three before starting to gulp down my drink and ask for another one to be bought over. The heat was really starting to build up now and my cousins had stopped eating their lunch to watch me in horror, crying.

My hands were trembling holding the wings as my body was threatening to go into shock. I had never felt an impact like this before and one of my cousins even asked me to stop eating them.

"Never!" I screamed as my battle cry.

It was then the waitress slinked over to our table.

"I told you they were hot." she said with a smirk on her face.

I just smiled sweetly at her through the tears and sweat.

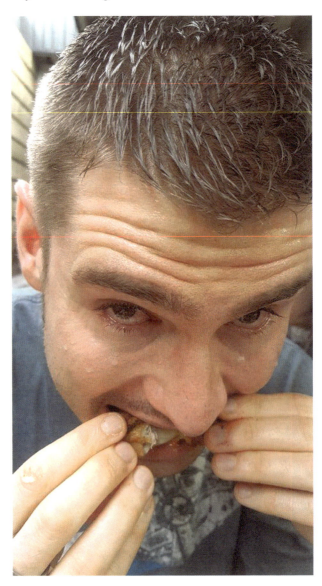

Now sometimes the only way out, is to go so far in.

I refused to be beaten. I stopped for a moment, so my body could adapt to the heat and used the sour cream sauce as a bath in which to soak my tongue between mouthfuls. The bowl of wings never seemed to end but finally I could start to see more bones than wings.

A very painful 25 minutes later and I had done it! I had finished the bowl of mega hog wings.

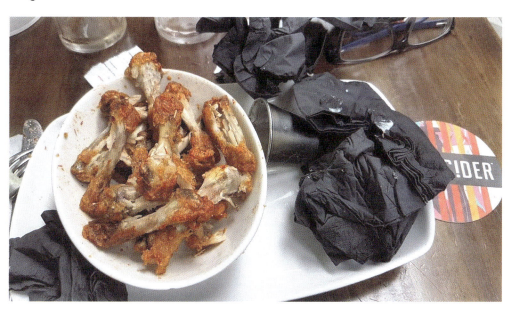

The same smarmy waitress came up to me after and said, "Well done. I have never seen anyone finish them before."

I found out after that the sauce was made with the Carolina Reaper chilli pepper, one of the hottest in the world mentioned earlier on. I can assure you I will not be ordering those wings again in a hurry.

It was only after finishing my wings that it dawned on me. I had ordered a spicy jalapeno burger for my main!

The New You

Now I need to warn you. You're going to get some jealous bitches out there once you have completed your own personal 'Shit Yourself Thin' program.

For example:

"No wonder your knees hurt, your too skinny. Got no shock absorbers! This is a picture of you sitting down!"

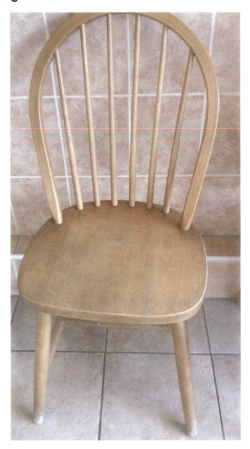

That was a text from my Mum while I was on my holiday in the US.

"You need to stop losing weight, you look like you have AIDS!"

That was another family member #awkward

But don't let the trolling get you down!

I even accidentally found myself flirting with the dentist the other day:

> "Have you lost weight Mr McNally?"
>
> "Erm, maybe." – I said seductively.
>
> "You have a very clean mouth. Must be all that flossing!"
>
> "I know." – I replied with a wink.

I didn't have the heart to tell him I didn't floss!

Back in 2015 I did a Masters in Strategic Business Management for a bit of a "laugh". Now do not get me wrong it was very tough trying to do that at the same time as my full-time job, side jobs and my social life and I was screaming blue murder while I was doing it.

It was such a good feeling however having done the regime to be able to attend my graduation with my partner and parents and get my photo taken.

You can really see where I have lost the weight around my face and neck.

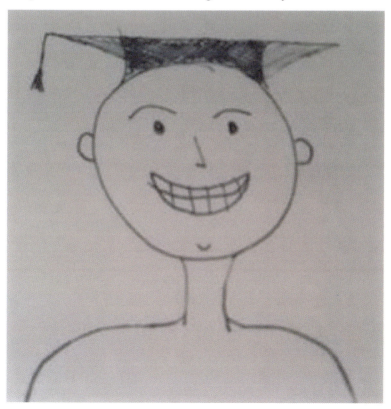

I used the Health Tracker on my phone to record my weight every week on a Monday evening. Based on my last check I had lost a total of 3.1 stone. Not bad I didn't think based on what I had done and where I have been.

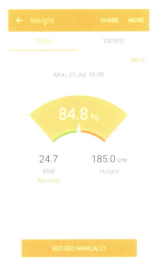

This diet plan/regime/torture method was never meant to be a long-term thing and I have now stopped. The reasons being that my mission has been accomplished. I lost weight was happy with that. However, there was something on the horizon coming which was harder than losing weight...keeping it off!!

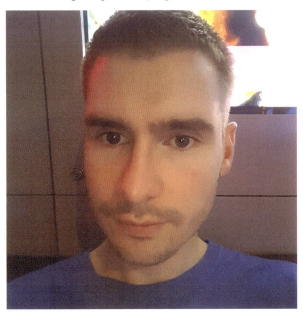

Above: Me in October 2017 staying thin!

Below: Me in July 2017 showing off my new sexy figure

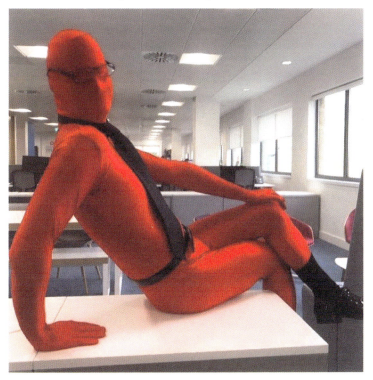

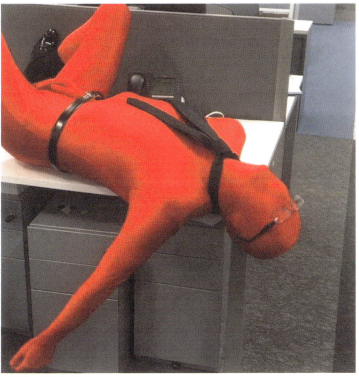

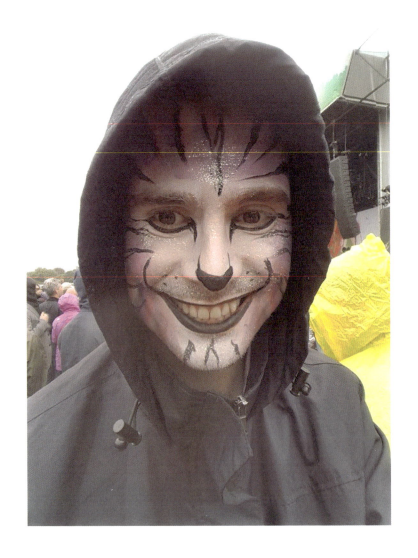

If I can do it, you can do it!

'Shit Yourself Thin'

#syst

By Joseph McNally

Printed in Great Britain
by Amazon